Contents

Dis-Ease

Middle English (in the sense 'lack of ease; inconvenience'): from Old French *desaise* 'lack of ease', from *des-* (expressing reversal) + *aise* 'ease'[1]

To place emphasis on the natural state of "ease" being imbalanced or disrupted. [2]

Dis: a Latin prefix meaning "apart," "asunder," "away," "utterly," or having a privative, negative, or reversing force.[3]

Introduction

I was diagnosed with prostate cancer, of which there are apparently some 27 varieties[4], on 1 July 2011. Given my cancer staging I opted for active surveillance, but on 12 October 2012 a second biopsy indicated my cancer had increased and become more aggressive. On December 7, 2012 I had a radical prostatectomy.

When I learned I had cancer I told my wife I was not going to write "The Book." First, I did not want to become identified with and by my disease. Christopher Hitchens said in his book *Mortality*: "Trying not to think with my tumour, which would not be thinking at all.[5]" So, if I may: Trying not to become my cancer, which would not be me at all. Second, autobiographical writing about life threatening illnesses can be maudlin, or saccharine, or melodramatic, or self-indulgent, or, is it possible, all the above. Third, the all-pervasive Oprah culture that insists public pseudo-psychological exposure is the means to healing and self-actualization is, at least to me, cheap entertainment. And fourth, while writing may be therapeutic for some, I do not write as a form of therapy. And yet, here we are.

So now you know what I am trying to avoid while writing *Dis-Ease*, but not what I would hope to accomplish. Well…I write in part to make meaning out of the jumble of experiences that make up my life and cancer surely jumbles things up. Also, I am quite willing and comfortable talking about prostate issues, something many men are not. So I write this not-a-book to make meaning and to communicate. Meaning and Communiqué. Simple as that.

What follows is not a systematic accounting of an illness and its treatment. It is rather a blog I wrote during the process, a collection of meditations[6] dealing with the very practical aspects and very personal implications of prostate cancer and treatments and some metaphysical musings motivated by what I was going through.

Before we begin, however, I need to state clearly that *I am not medically trained*. I am just a guy with prostate cancer trying to figure things out. What I have shared is what I have learned through reading, talking to medical staff and from Prostate Cancer UK.[7] If you have concerns about any aspect of prostate health and disease, please consult your doctor and do you own research.

The Case for Unintelligent Design

If you have a prostate, or love someone who has a prostate, sometime in the immediate or distant future you might become concerned. Here's why.

The prostate gland completely embraces the urethra, from the urethra's opening to the bladder at the top to the urethral sphincter at the bottom. Or another way of putting it, between the bladder and the urethral sphincter the urethra runs right through the middle of the prostate. Running across and adhering to the prostate are the cavernous nerves that control erections. Also touching the prostate, or in close touching distance of the gland, are the seminal vesicles, ejaculatory ducts, bladder and rectum. In other words, quite a bundle of stuff important to a man. When everything is working fine, all is well. But when the prostate becomes cancerous, as it does in one in six men, it's a real mess. Here's why.

During a radical prostatectomy the cavernous nerves must be peeled away and even if done successfully almost men will experience erectile dysfunction for weeks or months or even years. Some men will be impotent the rest of their lives. Also, external beam radiotherapy, brachytherapy, high intensity focused ultrasound (HIFU) and cryotherapy may damage the nerves and cause erectile dysfunction as well.

If a man opts for radical surgery, as I did, his libido will be unaffected and he will be able to have orgasms (with or without an erection), but he will not be able to ejaculate because the seminal vesicles and ejaculatory ducts will have been removed with the prostate. And radiotherapy, brachytherapy, HIFU and cryotherapy are more than likely going to reduce the amount of ejaculate.

All treatments affect the urethra, urethral sphincter and bladder which means most men will experience incontinence for weeks or months while others will have the condition for years. Finally, there is a small chance men will have problems with their rectum and defecating. So, treatment of the prostate gland can cause trouble with urinating, defecating, ejaculating and erections. All in all, the prostate is nothing less than a colossal design flaw.

All this prostate reality stirs in me some metaphysical wandering and wondering because at bottom line prostate cancer can force a man to reconsider his life and what it is to be a man, whether or not he survives the cancer or eventually dies. For example, early on in my journey with prostate cancer I got to thinking about me and God (and here substitute whatever metaphysical force or being you choose). Given the reality of the prostate gland there are only three things I could say about God. One, God doesn't exist. How could any supreme being create something so stupidly designed as the prostate gland?

Two, God is stupid. However, the very notion of a stupid supreme being is contrary to any and all reasonable definition of what a supreme being should be. So, we are back to proposition one: He/She/It doesn't exist.

Three, God exists but has a very questionable sense of humour. When in the history of our species men's life expectancy was 20 or 30 or 40 or even 50 years, the prostate was no problem at all. But now that men are living long past 60 years, the prostate is a real pain in the ass. Presumably a supreme being to which a day is like a thousand years and a thousand years is like a day, knew this was going to happen. If He/She/It didn't, we're back to the proposition that God is stupid, or as Woody Allen suggested:

> "The important thing, I think, is not to be bitter. You know, if it turns out that there is a God, I don't think that he's evil. I think that the worst you can say about him is that basically he's an underachiever."[8]

I found I was forced to at least consider the notion that Native Americans were right when they told stories about Coyote. In the Native American understanding of reality, life is endowed with the spirit of the First People and Coyote is one of the First People who lives on in human form. In mythologies and stories Coyote is a the Great Trickster, and as such he was also a Glutton, Lecher, Thief, Cheat, Outlaw, Spoiler, Loser, Clown, Survivor:

...you know, Coyote
is in the origin and all the way
through...he's the cause
of the trouble, the hard times
that things have...
Yes, he came so close
to having it easy.
But he said,

"Things are just too easy..."

(From *A Good Journey* by Simon Ortiz[9])

And:

Trickster's time
is not clicked off neatly
on round dials nor shadowed
in shifty digits:
he counts his changes slowly
and is not accurate.
He lives in his own mess of words,
his own burnt stew: he sees
when the singers are spread
and trapped by their songs,
numbed by the sounds of space
and reach their limit
so then can't hear the frozen music
circle above us like ravens or
like grubs flow into fleshy thrums
at their feet.
Trickster turns to wind,
Trickster turns to sand,
Trickster leaves you groping,
Trickster swings walking off
with your singer's tongue
left inaudible...
We see only his grey tail
bird-disguised
like a moving target
as he steals all the words
we ever thought
we knew.

(From *Lost Copper* by Wendy Rose[10])

Sometimes the jokes are funny and on Coyote himself, but often they are hard and on us:

> Deciding the cavernous nerves had to adhere to the prostate gland knowing that treatment would either burn or damage them thus leaving that all important organ limp while the libido soars;
>
> Putting the ejaculatory ducts so close to the prostate that any treatment will likely to lead to dry orgasms;
>
> Butting the prostate up against the urethral sphincter assuring that at least for a time a man will uncontrollably pass urine but not semen.

Presumably all that's pretty damn funny to a supreme being, regardless of His/Hers/Its name.

Still, I'm not bitter. The options seem clear:

> Option One: Learn to Laugh Through the Treatment;
>
> Option Two: Possibly Die.

Personally, I went with Option One. If Option One proves intolerable, there is always Option Two. But if you chose Option Two, there is no going back. And that's no laughing matter.

A friend on Facebook sent me the following:

> Three people were debating if God were an engineer what kind he would be. The first proposed he must be a mechanical engineer: Just look at the intricacy of bones and joints, the interplay of leverages.
>
> No, said the second, he's an electrical engineer: Look at the complexity of nerve signalling systems, the finely balanced voltages, the neural network computer that can actually learn.
>
> Both are wrong said the third: He's a civil engineer because only a civil engineer would lay a sewage pipe through a recreational area.

I loved it. I laughed out loud sitting all alone in my study. And I keep hearing laughter is good for me.

However, there is a danger that we are becoming a bit casual about prostate cancer. A significant number of men get prostate cancer so it is almost seen as normal. And often prostate cancer is benign and will just hang around until you get that heart attack. So no big deal. Not to worry. When I began telling people I was diagnosed with prostate cancer, I was struck by the number of people who said something like this:

> "Oh. Well that's pretty common and it probably won't hurt you. I mean most men have prostate cancer and don't even know it."

I am moved to share some hard facts the divine Great Civil Engineer has left with us, and which, I would suggest, reinforce the need for laughter.

According to Prostate Cancer UK:

> Prostate cancer kills one man every hour of every day.
>
> Over a quarter of a million men are living with the disease today.
>
> The number of men with the disease is rising at an alarming rate.
>
> It is predicted that by 2030 prostate cancer will be the most prevalent of all cancers in the UK.
>
> The best blood test for identifying prostate cancer is unreliable. Presently there is *no* test that can consistently tell who has the life threatening form of the disease.
>
> If prostate cancer is identified at a late stage, there is no cure.
>
> There are often no symptoms.
>
> Treatment of the disease can have a powerful impact on men's bodies and their psychological health. [11]

Over half of men will contract some form of prostate problem in their lifetime. That's the bad news, and while all these numbers, statistics and projections need to be taken very seriously, it would be wrong not to also say that things are improving. Research is advancing and treatments are improving. For example, when my father had prostate surgery, it was assumed that he would end up incontinent and impotent. He did. But looking at my prostate surgery I knew the odds were very low that I would experience long term incontinence. I've read and have been told that only 3%-5% or 4%-6% of men (depending on the treatment and who does the figuring) end up with long term incontinence - meaning longer than six months. And while the odds of impotence are greater, the medical people I have spoken to prefer to speak of erectile dysfunction, not the permanent condition of impotence.

Even better news is that if the disease is caught early men have every chance of surviving and living full lives. But the Great Civil Engineer is in the details. While we have more information, there is still so much we don't know, and this means that many men with prostate problems, if not most, will need to make decisions about their health and quality of life based on *not* knowing what might actually happen. Let me explain.

The PSA blood test, as noted above, is not all that reliable. The prostate gland produces a protein we called Prostate Specific Antigen (PSA) and all men have some PSA in their blood. An increase in the PSA level may indicate cancer, but it may not. Your level may rise because of your age, or benign prostate enlargement, or an infection, or because you've had an orgasm within three days of the test. As a general rule: *while one PSA blood test is not reliable, a pattern of tests results over several months may be important.*

But here's the dilemma. If your PSA is up, should you have a prostate biopsy, which in my experience was unpleasant but not painful?[12] The PSA rise might be an indication of cancer or it might be nothing. The only way to really tell is a biopsy, but statistics suggest that many men have unnecessary biopsies. If you do have a biopsy and you are diagnosed with cancer, they should give you your Gleason Score (the measurement of the aggressiveness of your cancer), the number of biopsy samples that were cancerous and the percentage of cancer cells in the affected samples, and after an MRI and a bone scan tell you whether or not it is likely that the cancer has spread to other parts of your body.

To further complicate matters, the all important Gleason Score is not as concrete a number as we would hope for. A Gleason Score is a *predictive measurement* indicating the probable state of the prostate cancer and its outcome. This measurement is based on the tumour's grade which is an indication of its aggressiveness. The grade suggests how far the tumour has deviated from healthy cells, thus grade 1 cells are very similar to the pattern of healthy cells while grade 5 cells are very irregular and disorganised. A Gleason Score is derived from the two most "prevalent organizational patterns" in the tumour, each pattern being assigned a number which are added together to get a final score. So a score of 5 + 3 has a Gleason Score of 8, where the 5 indicates the most common pattern of cells is also the most disorganised and distorted from healthy cells and the 3 signifies the least common pattern of cells which also has the least deviation from healthy cells. Thus a score of 5 + 3 is worse than a score of 3 + 5.[13]

It should also be noted that assigning grades to cancer cells is an *interpretive process*. A urologist physically looks down a microscope and judges how close a pattern of cells is to the Gleason images and gradings. Two different urologists might come up with two different gradings for the same tumour. For example, my first Gleason Score was 3 + 3 = 6 and my second was 4 + 3 = 7. One consultant suggested my score had not actually changed over the year between readings, but that the urologists interpreting the results came up with different conclusions.

Most urologists consider Gleason Scores of 5 or 6 to represent low-grade nonaggressive cancers, 7 intermediate and 8 or above to be high-grade aggressive cancers. But what of a score of 5 or 6? If the cancer is nonaggressive and localised in the prostate, it may stay that way until you peacefully die of old age. Or it may change in time. We just don't know. Do you play the odds or get the treatment? It's a very difficult question because any treatment will have a significant impact on your life. But if you play the odds and lose, you will more than likely die.

I personally set numerical limits over which I would take the next step on the journey. So, I decided if my PSA remained above 4 I would have a biopsy. It did and I had a biopsy. If my Gleason Score were above 6 I would undergo treatment, which after a year it was (my first score was 3 + 3, my second 4 + 3). And if treatment were called for, I would simply choose the one that seemed to offer the best results and was the less traumatic given my physical and psychological conditions. The medical staff and Prostate Charity UK have been great with me, but ultimately they couldn't tell me all that I wanted to know and they certainly didn't make decisions for me.
It's a game about urinating, defecating, sex, life and death. Welcome to the world where a sewage pipe runs through a recreational area.

What Did I Do to Deserve This?

When I went to the hospital to have my prostate removed, and after waiting three hours in Surgical Reception, I was ushered into a room with six cubicles and lots of equipment. It was in one of these cubicle that I talked to the anaesthetist, the surgeon and changed into my hospital gown. Since all the curtains were drawn, I could not see who was in the other cubicles. However, I could hear them quite easily.

In the cubicle to my right was a man having a catheter jammed down his penis through his urethra and into his bladder in preparation for surgery. (For female readers, men do not like having things jammed into their penises. Even thinking about it makes us cringe. Test it. Talk to a man about having something jammed into his penis and watch his face.[14]) His way of dealing with this intrusion was humour and feigning, in my opinion, scientific and technological interest in the procedure. It seemed to work for him.

In the next cubicle was an 81 year old man. I knew he was 81 because he kept telling everyone who entered his cubicle that he was 81. He smoked heavily throughout his life, but had quit years ago and was thus bemused by the fact that now at 81 surgeons wanted to deal with the "shadow on his lung." He was also angry because no one told him he would have to spend the night in the hospital. His blood pressure was high, too high for an operation, which didn't surprise him since he was scheduled for surgery, there was no one to pick him up the next day, his cell phone was running out of juice and his house was flooded.

Next to him was another man, also having a catheter inserted in preparation for surgery. What his particular illness was that demanded surgery I did not know, but he said this in a quiet somewhat weary and sad voice: "What did I do to deserve this?"

How many ill or injured human beings have asked that question? I would guess most. It may be instinctive.

The immediate implication of this question is that our physical condition is caused by our behaviour. Sometimes this is true. It is not a stretch to assume that a cancerous tumour in the lungs of an 81 year old man was caused by years of heavy smoking. But such obvious and well known causal relationships between our bodies and our behaviour were not at the heart of the man's angst. The question assumed that our physical condition is *caused by our moral behaviour*. Or put another way, our bodily state is determined by our morality. And, of course, there is more. Such a notion also implies that God, or the Gods, or Fate, or The Force or Whatever is, through disease and injury, punishing us for our immorality. Indeed, the idea of a causal relationship between body and morality demands the presence of a judging agent of some kind. Nonetheless, it is all nonsense.

Firsts, there is no causal connection between our bodies and our morality. There is no amount of immoral behaviour that caused the man in the cubicle to have a disease that required surgery. And the reverse is true. No amount of virtuous behaviour would have protected him from his illness.

Second, if your interpretation of reality and your theology do lead you to conclude that God, or the Gods, or Fate, or The Force or Whatever punishes you with illness/injury and rewards you with good health based on your moral behaviour, then you really do need to seriously rethink things. I would suggest that if there were a God, or the Gods, or Fate, or The Force or Whatever that punishes and rewards in this way She, He, It or They would not be worthy of your time and certainly not your worship. In this regard, for those of you who are concerned about God, or the Gods, or Fate, or The Force or Whatever, a little but important book by Gustavo Gutierrez entitled *On Job: God-Talk and the Suffering of the Innocent*[15] may help (a book I recommend to the religious and nonreligious both). Gutierrez asks this question at the very beginning of the book:

> Can human beings have a disinterested faith in God – that is, can they believe in God without looking for rewards and fearing punishment? Even more specifically: Are human beings capable, in the midst of unjust suffering, of continuing to assert their faith in God and speak of God without expecting a return?[16]

The word "disinterested" is difficult in this context. At first glance it implies having a faith or worldview that is disconnected and indifferent. Indeed, turning to the numerous online dictionaries we find one definition to be: not interested and indifferent. But the word also means: unbiased by personal interest or advantage; not influenced by selfish motives.[17]

What Gutierrez means by a disinterested faith in God, and I would add a disinterested interpretation of reality, is that such a faith or interpretation should not be based on the selfish fear of punishment and hope of reward, but on the value of the relationship itself. We love God, or Life, not because it may harm us or reward us, but because God and Life are worthy of love. Or, being in a truthful relationship with God, or Life, is meaningful in and of itself. Put more basically: I do not love my wife because she may punish or reward me, but because she is worthy of love.

Finally, there is something deeply sad about the question: "What did I do to deserve this?" I say this because we all have been bad at times and we all know it of ourselves, and when we ask this question we do so knowing this about our lives. The question, therefore, indicates a state of confusion, angst and existential despair: I know I have been bad at times, but *what* did I do that was *so* bad that I *deserve* this? If am being punished, tell me what my sin was, for then I might more easily cope. It's a rather Kafkaesque moaning that will never be answered. Sometimes we just get sick.

The Movements of a Dis-Ease

When I had my gall bladder removed years ago it was a fairly simple process, or so it seems now looking back through the filters of time and memory. Before the surgery I had been in pain for quite some time and was more than glad to be anesthetized and have the surgeons take the damn thing out. What followed was a few days in hospital and recovery at home, no complications and no fuss. The worst I had to consider beyond recovery was occasional heartburn. However, this time around it was different. Given the nature of prostate problems the process is better approached in movements, and while each movement calls for a particular physical and emotional response, the transition between movements is equally demanding.

First Movement: Numbers and Anxiety

My back landed me in bed for several months and my GP, whom I very much like, trust and respect, insisted on a PSA test saying something like: "When men your age have persistent back pain I like to check their PSA level." I let the comment about my age pass, but as it turned out she was right to run the PSA. The initial results indicated my PSA was very high.

As this movement began, these were the numbers that began to change my life:

> 14;
> 11.2;
> 9.6.
> PSA = Prostate Specific Antigens, an enzyme produced by the glandular cells in the prostate. Levels are expressed in nanograms per millilitre or ng/mL. A good prostate level is 2 ng/mL or 3ng/mL.

There is nothing so reassuring as the concreteness of numbers. Unfortunately, though we all agree that 3 + 3 = 6, it's not necessarily so when diagnosing prostate problems. Truth is, the experts don't always know what the numbers mean. In reality you have to make decisions based on numbers that lack their commonly expected certainty. High PSA numbers are not good, but they may be elevated because you had an infection, or due to your age, or because you had an orgasm within three days of the test. They may indicate an enlarged prostate that is troublesome but benign, or a nonaggressive cancer that will remain so for many years, or an aggressive cancer that will surely kill you sooner rather than later. Regardless, you have to decide what to do. Get it wrong one way and you go through unpleasant and/or painful life changing procedures you never needed. Get it wrong the other way and you die. 3 + 3 may equal nothing or it may equal everything. Numbers and anxiety are intimates in the world of prostate problems.

After nine months of blood tests I had decided that a PSA level of 4 or above on the next test would trigger a biopsy. The urologist seemed genuinely relieved I had a plan and had made a decision. On the day of the procedure urology was running an hour behind schedule and for all that time I imagined I was about to have an experience akin to the worse nightmare in an Edgar Allan Poe story. Waiting is difficult. My anxiety had more to do with the fear of pain than the more abstract, at that time, fear of cancer. I doubt anyone believes they have cancer until they are told that indeed they do. Even assuming the worst, because your glass is always half empty, is not the same as knowing the worst. In any event, the biopsy wasn't all that bad. Unpleasant, yes, but not painful, though I must say you need to leave your dignity at the door (essentially a stranger inserts a camera and a needle gun into your rectum).

The day I met my cancer the urology department was running an hour and a half behind schedule. Again it was all about numbers and anxiety. The anxiety swirled around the thought of entering a reality where the unbelievable by necessity, for only necessity can force this kind of transformation, becomes believable. As I waited to be told in which reality I would pitch my tent, I knew the odds were that I had cancer. All but one of the indicators pointed that way:

> High PSA (should be low);
> Low free PSA (PSA in the blood binds to proteins so you want a high percentage of free or unbound proteins) ;
> Significant change in PSA in a year;
> Prostate was not enlarged (an enlarged prostate gland can cause PSA to rise);
> Family history (both my father and grandfather had prostate cancer).

When the moment comes, tangible numbers with ambiguous meanings and multi-faceted anxiety cast shadows. The only way through is acceptance.

When I was told I had cancer I believe my response was: “I’m not surprised. What is my Gleason Score?”

A Gleason Score indicates the aggressiveness of a cancer. 5 or 6 is nonaggressive, 7 is ambiguous and 8 and above is aggressive. My score was 6. But even this friendly number demanded companionship. Within days I had a full body bone scan and a pelvic MRI to determine if my cancer was localized or had metastasized.

Here are the numbers that end the First Movement:

T1 (Cancer localized in prostate)
Gleason 3+3 (Nonaggressive cancer)
1/14 Cores (Number of samples cancerous)
10% (Percentage of cancerous cells in sample)
26.5ml (Gland size)
N0 (Bone scan clear)
M0 (Pelvic MRI clear)

All those numbers seemed so actual, so earthed. However…If the statisticians are right, and surely they are, that most men who undergo biopsies and treatments never needed them and that they would have died of that infamous heart attack in noble old age never knowing their prostates were diseased, then what do I do with my numbers? You can see how the complacency surrounding prostate cancer so easily sets in, how men and their loved ones so quickly and, well, extraordinarily, trumpet their up-coming broken heart. On the other hand, if the statisticians happened to be wrong in my particular case and my specific prostate, then it is not reputations that are lost, but my life.

Second Movement: Coping with Reality and Watching the Numbers

I met with an oncologist, a urologist and an oncology nurse to receive the above numbers. It was the second high stake appointment I had to wait on, anticipate, imagine, fear, and participate in (more were to come, each one raising the stakes). How do I describe the emotional response to and engagement with this process? There is no escaping the moment when the information you both need and fear is spoken. No matter that every fibre of your being wants either to delay the utterance or spur it on, there is a precise moment which you cannot control but nonetheless changes your life. It is a moment of reality, or rather a moment of reality creation. The words "you do not have cancer" send you in one direction. The words "you have cancer" send you in another. But either way, the reality in which you live has changed.

I had decided that if my Gleason Score were less than 7 and the cancer were localized I would forgo treatment and instead watch, wait and live with my disease. Treatment is no joking matter. Putting aside the trauma of the treatment you choose (they are all tough going), you will experience incontinence (though the odds are you will overcome it) and erectile dysfunction (the odds of recovery here are less good). With the 6 and the two 0's (from the MRI and bone scan) in my mind, I walked out of the oncologist's office feeling elated. Before the utterance "You have cancer" I would never have been pleased by these numbers. But after the utterance "You have cancer," well, I couldn't have asked for better numbers. Yes, I had cancer, but it was nonaggressive and localized. Bring on that old man's heart attack sometime in the undisclosed future.

All agreed I would pursue a strategy of active surveillance, which means blood tests every three months and a biopsy, MRI scan and bone scan once a year if necessary. It's simple. If you can live peacefully with cancer in your body, acknowledging that you will have some bad days– you have cancer, after all! – then active surveillance is the way to go. After all, as we keep hearing, prostate cancer can lie low for years until that day you die peacefully in your favourite chair a contented old man. Surveillance until you die of something else. Or the watching can be short-lived. Just no way of knowing. Statistics are one thing. Guarantees are another, and there are no guarantees.

While I doubt a day went by when I did not think about my cancer, I more than not lived peacefully with my dis-ease. Yes, contradictory but manageable. I did become anxious at the time of each blood test simply because a change in the numbers paints in broad brush strokes your future. Active surveillance pits the fragility of hope against the insistence of numbers (the hope being, of course, that you will be among the lucky with a relatively benign prostate cancer for years). These are the numbers that undermined my hope:

8.2;

8.8;
10.64;
10.98; and
11.27.

As each number went up, my hope went down. When my PSA hit 11.27 I was sent for another MRI which showed a lesion on my prostate. From there it was a no-brainer; another biopsy, the results of which showed an increase in the number of samples with cancerous cells and an increase in my Gleason Score to 4 + 3. That was that. I had decided long ago that a Gleason of 7 or above would necessitate treatment. So much for hope and the comfort of statistics.

Third Movement: Technology, Chemistry and Radical Vulnerability

In the Third Movement numbers begin to fade in importance as the pure physicality of Western medicine becomes dominant.

It is here that you embrace radical vulnerability as you turn your body, your health and perhaps your life over to strangers who possess medical knowledge and skills you cannot understand. Here you are not a great warrior fighting your cancer. You are the epitome of vulnerability and trust.

The point is this. Western medicine can improve or even save our lives, but the intrusion of technology and chemistry into our bodies comes at a very high price.

The first thing I became aware of after my radical prostatectomy was being in bed in intensive care with the curtains drawn. A young woman came through the curtains, talked rapidly and in a friendly way, I assume about my medical situation, but then stopped suddenly in mid-sentence and said: "Do you remember me?" I did not, but said yes anyway. I wasn't distressed and wasn't all that aware of my body. I simply had no idea where I was or what was going on. Yes, seemed as good as no.

I later learned that when I was awoken after surgery, the surgeon called my wife to tell her the operation was completed, handed me his mobile phone so I could talk with her, that she asked if my face and eyes were swollen,[18] that I asked the anaesthetist if that were indeed so and grunted something back into the phone. I was then transferred to intensive care where I was introduced to the nursing staff and an anaesthetist (in fact the rapidly talking young woman). I remembered absolutely none of this.

When the anaesthetist left me I examined my body (I remember nothing of what she said to me at that meeting behind drawn curtains). I had, of course, numerous intravenous lines, which I believe the nurses called "taps." I had a tap on the outside of my left hand, another in the side of my left wrist just below my thumb and a third in the artery of my left inside wrist. In my right forearm was a fourth tap. Coming out of my left side was a drainage tube that sucked blood and other fluids from my abdomen into a small clear bag pinned to my hospital gown. In my penis was a tube running through my urethra into my bladder. The catheter bag with bloody urine hung on the side of the bed. I knew that I had had a tube inserted in my nose down into my stomach and a larger tube inserted in my throat to help me breathe, but both had been removed before I became fully aware of my surroundings. My entire abdomen was both bloated and swollen. The bloating was the result of air being pumped into my abdomen to increase the working space for the robot. I was told my abdominal muscles would be sore for some time due to the considerable air pressure. The swelling was due to the cutting and probing of the actual surgery. I had six incisions which were sutured and covered with a clear glue (and a seventh where the suction tube was inserted.) Each wound was swollen and bruising was already evident A tube and bag containing a clear liquid hanging on a pole next to the bed were attached to the tap in my right forearm. The tap in my left artery was attached to a machine beside my head. Numerous colourful numbers continually flashed. I was in considerable pain. I felt like I had been assimilated by the Borg[19]. And I knew it could have been worse.

This eventful day had begun in the surgical waiting lounge where I sat for three hours reading *Arguably* by Christopher Hitchens. This was my second time waiting in this lounge and I was determined not to become frozen with anxiety as I waited for the call. Ten days earlier I was unable to read simply because I could not concentrate. After a four hour wait the surgery was cancelled by the surgeon saying a replacement assistant was not "fit for purpose" and was "really terrible." He thus refused to operate. I was grateful for his honesty and his unwillingness to proceed, but the disappointment was visceral.

I was eventually ushered into another room containing six beds with the curtains drawn. There I changed into two hospital gowns (the second to hide my butt), surgical leggings and slippers. First came the anaesthetist who looked like he was twelve years old. He explained that I would be put to sleep and wheeled into the theatre. There I would be strapped safely to the bed which would be tilted down so my head was below my feet. Given that I would be in that position for four to five hours, it was likely that my face and eyes would become swollen, as would my brain which in turn might cause confusion. During the operation my brain would be monitored to determine the depth of my unconsciousness as the robot manipulated by the surgeon some distance away from me would cut into my body. Six ports would be inserted to enable easy access for the robot. My abdomen would be filled with air to facilitate the surgery. The anaesthetist was a pleasant and self-confident person who left me feeling safe, but nonetheless I was worried. My surgery was taking place on a Friday afternoon and I had read that one should avoid surgery on Mondays and Fridays so I asked him if he was running off to the pub when the operation was completed. He laughed and said the whole team was on duty until at least eight. This reassured me.

Next came the surgeon who explained the surgical procedure pleasantly but soberly. He showed me a drawing someone had made of my prostate which indicated where the cancer was located. He seemed slightly concerned about the location of the cancer cells, but I didn't ask why. He explained the risks and reminded me of the consequences of treatment: possible long term incontinence and erectile dysfunction. I told him I was fully aware of these possibilities. He asked if I had any erectile dysfunction in the past and when I said I had not, he said: "That's in your favour but your erections will never be as good." Such is life. He also said that if my lymph nodes "looked dodgy" he would take samples for biopsy. As it turned out he took samples. He was a tall man with big hands, so big in fact I thought it better the robot would be rooting around inside me. When he had finished and began leaving the confines of my curtained cubicle I called out: "Have a good afternoon!" He turned, laughed, said something I did not hear and left.

This was all about steel, plastic and chemicals. I would be forced into unconsciousness and made completely vulnerable. Plastic tubing would keep the chemicals coming. A machine would monitor my level of consciousness, heart rate, blood pressure, blood oxygenation, etc. The surgeon would never touch me. A robot would cut me inside and out. My role? Simply to put my trust in these strangers and hand over my body to be sliced and diced. It is perhaps not surprising that while the anaesthetist and surgeon were friendly, I nonetheless subconsciously attempted to introduce some semblance of human connection through the use of humour.

I wanted two contradictory things from the surgical team. I wanted my procedure to be routine for them, almost as if they were on a factory assembly line knocking off yet another operation. I wanted them to have done what they were going to do to me a thousand times before. But I also wanted them, however fleetingly and tenuously, to have a clear sense that I was a person who deserved their full attention. I wanted them to remember I was unique and vulnerable. I wanted them to care for me. I would never see either the anaesthetist or surgeon again[20].

It may be the case that the surgery saved my life, but the impact of the procedure was not insignificant. For several hours after the operation I felt like I had been hit by a train. The next day things improved and I felt like I had been run over by a truck. I found it difficult to look at my abdomen: the swelling, the seven wounds, the bruising, the tube running out of my body to a bag attached to my hospital gown. I looked and felt fragile. I was given pills, injections and numerous bags draining fluid into my body. I had only a vague notion of the purpose of the chemicals being dripped, injected and swallowed into my body. I did know that chemicals can distort your perception of reality which in turn can increase your sense of vulnerability. At one point while in hospital I saw a black spot on the corridor floor moving towards me but never getting any closer. While in intensive care my memory of being treated for nausea has me clearly sitting in a chair in the middle of the room when in fact I was next to my bed at the end of the room. When I had my gall bladder out as evening came I told my wife it was time for me to "go to the night place." At night under the influence of the drugs the ward was transformed and I felt as though I really was going to a different place. In my experience you just have to ride these things out and trust the people around you.

I had concerns during those first couple of days. I had to avoid nausea. I had to avoid constipation. I had to eat with no appetite. I had to watch my bloody urine. I had to sit up. I had to walk. I had to sleep. I had to hope nothing would go wrong. I had to give it time. I had to wait four weeks before hearing if the cancer had migrated from my prostate gland. I had to remain positive. I had to do my best, while all the time wanting to disappear from myself.

The surgery was completed by five on Friday afternoon. On Saturday afternoon the drainage tube was removed from my side. This as I knew from my gall bladder operation can be a *very* painful procedure. I was determined this time to keep my mouth tightly shut to muffle any scream into a growl. I asked Harry the nurse if he had a technique, say three deep breaths with the tube being pulled out on the third exhaling. He looked at me with a slight smile and said: “You’ve done this before. We do these things so often we can forget what it’s like for the patient. I’ll do it anyway you want.” As it turned out the removal was not as painful as my first experience, but the feeling of the tube trying to pull your insides out with its removal really does make you want to scream. It is simply something you should not have to feel.

On Sunday I became nauseous and the fast talking anaesthetist started hanging bags from poles. When the first two didn’t work she hung a third bag of magic, looked me in the eyes and said: “This *will* stop you feeling sick, but it will also make you feel very dizzy.” The words said what they needed to say, but the look said: “This is strong stuff!” She was right on all three counts, and as the chemical dripped through the tap on my forearm I had a moment of anxiety as I felt the drug affecting my body. Talk about trust.

On Monday morning at 8:30 the team of three consultants released me. I had had a nightmare of a night and was inclined to stay in the hospital. I had only taken very short walks and had only progressed to the “hit by truck” stage. While not unfriendly, the consultant who spoke simply said that another day in hospital was another day I was vulnerable to catching an infection of some kind. He wanted me to go home. Good for me and good for the hospital. And throughout this short conversation he had and air of slight indifference. The job was done. There were no apparent complications. Be gone. Fair enough.

Once I was released, the nurse removed my taps, and though they are but small intrusions, and though this will sound melodramatic, with the removal of each tap I felt more human. It felt good to have all the taps and tubes removed, with the exception of the catheter which I would take home with me.

I left the hospital as 5:30 p.m. - yes, it took the hospital the full day to process my release. And with the worst taxi ride of my life the Third Movement ended.

Fourth Movement: Ugly Body, Pain and Catheter Care

The taxi driver helped me out of the taxi. Nice man. It was obvious I wasn't for this world. I can't tell you how great it was getting into my own bed. Both my wife and I felt a certain relief, relief not that "it" was over, but that we had survived the surgery and hospitalization and could move on to the next phase.

The challenge of the Fourth Movement was to make peace with my body, deal with my pain and take care of the catheter I brought home with me. My abdomen was bloated, bruised and painful to touch. I say more about this in *My George W. Bush Emotional Strategy for Coping with Dis-Ease*, but suffice it to say here that for a few days I didn't want to touch or look at myself. This, of course, passed. But for a few days things were more than difficult. I wanted very little to do with my body.

I was in considerable pain which was understandable and expected. I had excellent care at the hospital, but I was surprised that they sent me home with only paracetamol and ibuprofen for pain management. Neither did the job during that first week so I emailed my GP and she put me on co-codamal. My GP has been a life saver more than once. Pain lets us know when something is wrong but it also retards our healing.

I struggled with the pain and like so many in my generation I was, am, ambiguous about taking pain medication. "Being a man" is to endure pain, and even though doctors and nurses have been telling me for years that the body heals better when not having to fight pain all the time, I still take the meds reluctantly. My message to others: take the damn pain medication.

I was given careful instructions before I checked out of the hospital about how to care for my catheter. The catheter tube came out of my penis attached to a leg bag which was held in place on my thigh by a Velcro strap. The tube and bag were both clear plastic so you could see the urine and oftentimes blood easing its way into the bag. I also had a night bag, that I hung from the bed frame, with a long tube that attached to the bottom of the leg bag so I could sleep through the night and not worry about having to go to the toilet to empty the bag.

My instructions included drinking a lot of fluids and keeping the inner tip of my penis as clean as possible. The last thing you want is an infected penis. At the beginning sleeping and walking were a challenge. I had to sleep on my back so as not to get tangled up in the catheter and thus pull it unnecessarily. Moving and tugging the catheter tube was not scream out loud painful, but it was for me very uncomfortable, a stinging weird feeling that I really didn't like. Half the challenge was psychological, not physical. When I walked from room to room in the house and then outside, the tube would bend and pull with each stride. On the third day I told myself to stop thinking about it and accept that this was my life for another ten days. End of story.

Bottom line, it is not the end of the world to have a catheter in for two weeks. You just have to adjust. I was not bothered at all with emptying the leg bag several times a day and the night bag in the morning. It's just urine. My emotions did slide up and down depending on whether the urine was clear or bloody. I knew blood was common at this stage but every time I had a couple of days of clear urine followed by a few hours of bloody urine I became upset. There were two things to watch out for: blood clots and excessive bleeding. I was told blood clots meant I needed to call my district nurse or get to the hospital. Excessively bloody urine, again hospital or nurse. What excessive bloody urine would look like was somewhat of a mystery to me – I mean how different would excessive be from what I was experiencing? In the end, however, I never called a taxi to head back to the hospital, though on a couple of occasions I thought about calling the district nurse or emailing my GP.

In addition to living with the catheter my other major job was getting up and walking. It's the same old story. Walk enough to encourage healing, don't walk so much that you discourage healing. I did my best, but for the first week I was very reluctant to go outside simply because I wasn't sure how to manage the catheter, leg bag and underwear. I did everything I could to avoid tugging on that damn tube (I suspect, no I am sure, other men are much more manly about this than I was!).

My wife was given compassionate leave to stay home with me that first week out of hospital. A friend of ours in California, whose husband had gone through the same operation, emailed to say that it was important for my wife to be home that first week. We thought that a bit dramatic. It wasn't. From drying my legs after a shower (I couldn't bend over enough to reach my legs for several days), putting on my socks and shoes, preparing meals, encouraging me to walk and just being there, her presence was essential. (Our California friend's husband had the same problem with bags and underwear while walking so simply put the catheter bag in a small carrier bag which he held in his hand. Apparently he got a couple of strange looks from children, but it was much more comfortable.)

Ten days at home before the catheter was removed. Catheter care, walking and pain medications. I wasn't motivated to read, but could watch TV. I learned something of importance that week. I do not want to become a person who watches daytime TV. It really isn't good for you.

On the tenth day, after having the catheter for two weeks, I went to my local hospital to have the objectionable thing removed and thus began the Fifth Movement.

Fifth Movement: Man-Diapers and Pelvic Floor Exercises.

I was actually excited to go to the hospital on that tenth day. The joke is that the appointment to remove the catheter is the appointment no man is late for. I was early.

My oncology nurse is great. Before actually removing the catheter he showed me two large packages. The first was a pack of man-diapers. I call them man-diapers because it helps me feel better about the whole thing. He called them by some medical term which I didn't quite hear. I just looked at him and then said: "Oh you mean diapers." He laughed. The second package contained pads that you place in your underwear. He showed me both the man-diapers and the pads and explained that for the next few days I would not only need a man-diaper but a man-diaper with a pad because of my loss of bladder control. It sounded a bit sobering but hey, I was there to get the catheter removed so I took the news in good spirits.

The catheter that runs through your penis into your bladder is held in place by filling a small balloon at the end of the tube in the bladder with a saline solution. My oncology nurse had me lie on an examination table and he pulled the saline solution out of the balloon with a syringe. He then said he was going to withdraw the catheter, which only took a couple of seconds. It was not painful, though it did sting the inner tip of my penis. He had warned me that when he pulled the catheter out I would urinate and he placed paper towels between my legs. And so I did. He then asked me to put on my man-diaper. For whatever reason I experienced no embarrassment. Why? Because there is nothing to be embarrassed about. First, it's a medical issue. Second, my oncology nurse was so professional, nonchalant and friendly about the whole procedure it all seemed quite normal, normal that is under the circumstances.

I was asked to drink a lot of water and hang around for a couple of hours to make sure I could urinate. There is a seeming contradiction here. You wear a man-diaper because you have lost bladder control and yet you can't leave the hospital until you demonstrate you can urinate. Treatment for prostate cancer can cause incontinence and bladder retention. While I needed protection because I might urinate uncontrollably, I also needed to be able to urinate when I wanted to.

As it turned out, I only wore the man-diapers for two days and I suspect I could have abandoned them after the first. I used pads in my underwear for a few weeks, and again I probably could have stopped using those earlier but for my insecurity. I was fortunate, but not unusual.

In addition to man-diapers and pads the oncology nurse also gave me medication to aid me in having and maintaining erections. In my case it was Cialis® (tadalafil). He started me on two 10mg tablets each week and told me to take the meds but to expect no results. He was definitely right. For the first time in my life I have experienced sexual excitement with no reaction at all from my penis. Can't say I'm pleased, but it is what I expected and does tickle some intellectual pondering. Time will tell.

I continue to do my pelvic floor exercises, or Kegel exercises if you are in the U.S. I take long walks. I have watched the extensive bruising on my body fade. I have rejoiced as the pain receded. My energy is returning. I feel the flutter of creativity. I am reading and writing again. I can clean the house, though I must be careful not to strain my abdominal muscles. I keep going while not overdoing it. I think I see a light at the end of the tunnel.

Sixth Movement: Simply Live

For me prostate cancer and treatment have been a series of beginnings, endings and beginnings. I began with a high PSA which led to a biopsy which ended in a diagnosis of cancer. With that ending began active surveillance. When active surveillance ended surgery began. When surgery was completed hospital after care began. When my time in hospital ended the slow healing, walks and catheter care at home began. With the ending of the catheter regime began the pelvic floor exercises to regain bladder control and taking Cialis® to encourage erections. I am now beginning the Sixth Movement which will entail a year of blood tests to ascertain if any cancer cells were missed. But any way you look at it the Sixth Movement is simply to live.

The Handover

The hospital's shift handover took place between 8:00 and 8:30 each morning and evening. The head nurse from the shift ending would "hand over" the cases, which is to say the patients, to the head nurse of the shift beginning. They would stand at the end of my bed and talk *about* me. Actually, that's not quite accurate. They talked about my *condition*. How could it be otherwise? They didn't know me and weren't going to get to know me outside my illness and treatment. The handover was not about me, it was about passing on facts, charts and observations. I do not mean to imply that they ignored me. On the contrary, the new nurse would introduce himself or herself and often make eye contact during the handover. Except for an initial "Hello," I would just lie there saying nothing. My role was to be *The Body* with *The Disease*, which I did with consummate integrity.

After the ward handover was completed, the head nurse returned to me and explained that she or he was going to give me a quick look-over. First the handover, then the look-over. She or he first examined my toes, heals and ankles for swelling and any sign of bed sores. Then she or he would tell me to roll over onto one side and then the other to examine my bare back and bottom. I was exposed and helpless and followed her or his every instruction to the letter. Of course I did. But why did I acquiesce so easily?

Years ago when my wife and I were discussing the possibility of marrying, I told her that if she wanted me to do something it was best not to command me to do it. It is not that I particularly object to women or wives issuing commands, but rather that I have always had a delicious resistance to anyone commanding me to do anything. There are all sorts of ways to get me to do things, but commanding is not one of them. However, in the hospital, having been cut open, having had some of my innards cut apart and sewed back together and other parts completely removed, I not only obeyed commands, I welcomed them.

Interestingly, during the handover and look-over I did not feel objectified, though I did sense that such a possibility was waiting in the wings. It was vitally important to me that the new team got the information they needed to care for me. However, there was something more going on and that something more had a lot to do with my readiness to comply. The handover was not simply about data sharing and assimilation. After a twelve hour shift with one or two nurses caring for me, I had formed an embryonic relationship with them which was grounded in four essentials:

> Professional knowledge;
> Performance skills;
> Mutual cooperation; and
> Genuine trust.

I wanted those nonfactual uncharted experiences of virtual, but not quite, relationships that impacted my disease and treatment to also be somehow magically handed over. There is more to illness and healing than technology and chemistry. I needed to assume that the new team would be both able and willing to help me immediately. I didn't want to be invited to their daughter's wedding or to exchange Christmas cards, but I did want to trust that they could do their job and, despite the fact that I was a "patient," that they would see me and treat me as one of them: People.

Truthfully, this time around I was very fortunate. The medical staff, with the exception of one nurse who wasn't so much insensitive and stupid as preoccupied and sluggish, were excellent. They effectively balanced the need for objectivity towards my condition (which required knowledge, decision making and action) and sensitivity about my condition (which included pain, fear and radical vulnerability). This has not always been the case. When I had my gall bladder removed the surgeon who did the deed revealed himself to be extremely rude. Interestingly, during our pre-operation discussion in his office he was wonderful, describing without rush and with friendliness what he was going to do and why. But after the surgery, on the ward with his flock of students following in his wake, he made it clear that I had become a non-being. I was data. I was completed business. I was less than a rock. When I voiced a concern about my recovery, his initial indifference followed quickly by obvious annoyance were so pronounced that I would have fallen over but that I was already lying down. As he and his disciples rushed off, as if they had watched too many episodes of *ER*, one of the chosen remained behind and without saying the words "I'm sorry" nonetheless apologised. And there was the surgical consultant I met for my lower back problem. His so few words, voluminous body language and exposing open office door shouted that he had little or no interest in me and was unwilling or unable to grant me even a rudimentary respect. After the appointment I emailed my GP: “He may be an excellent consultant and surgeon but he should be kept away from patients who are awake.”

The relationship between vulnerability, trust and obedience is interesting. In the context of surgery and hospitalisation vulnerability is profound, and that very profundity demands both trust in and obedience to the medical experts. Trust has to be assumed, unless experience demands a reappraisal. (Having said that, I’m not sure I would have had the emotional and physical energy the first few days after surgery to mistrust anyone anyway.) Given the depth of patient vulnerability, obedience is only logical. We turn our bodies, and sometimes our lives, over to strangers with knowledge and expertise inaccessible and foreign to us, and once turned over we probably would not survive without their continued knowhow and care. Obviously, we can disobey, but to do so could be counterproductive and perhaps dangerous. Given the demands of illness we place before strangers our radical vulnerability which in turn necessitates that we trust and obey them. And it goes without saying that our trust and obedience assume these medical strangers are themselves trustworthy, but that is for another time.

The Indifferent Universe and Me

On January 4, 2013, exactly four weeks after my radical prostatectomy, I was told that my cancer had not spread beyond my prostate gland. Once again it was all about the numbers. My final pathology looks like this:

3+4
pT2c
N0
M0.

The 3+4 is my over all Gleason Score (aggressiveness of the cancer). They thought it might be 4+3, which would have been a big difference. But the 3+4 indicates the cancer was not as aggressive as they thought it might be.

The pT2c means this: the lower case p means the prostate has been removed; the T2 means the cancer was located in the gland (probably would be T1 in the U.S.); the lower case c means there were "clear margins," which in turn means the tissue that surrounded the prostate was cancer free.

N0 means my lymph nodes are cancer free and the M0 means my bones are cancer free.

There is a small "but" however, which is often the case. There is always a chance that a microscopic bit of cancer migrated beyond the gland that even the final pathology didn't pick up. So, for the next year I will have four PSA tests, the following year two PSA tests and after that one PSA a year for the rest of my life. However, to worry about this possibility would be perverse. All this means I am a very fortunate boy. And, of course, my good fortune got me thinking.

Imagine for a moment that standing next to me is a small child who also has a life threatening cancer (this is a very common mind exercise pitting the child's innocent life against my tarnished life). Imagine next that the small child, despite the confident prayers, the fevered prayers, the propositional prayers and the what-the-hell-I-might-as-well-give-it-a-try prayers, dies of her illness. It is important to recognize that "prayer," as understood and utilized in this context, assumes that God will or will not intervene in human suffering of all kinds, whether caused by natural events or human behaviour.

When I imagine this, I become angry as I react to the injustice of her death and my survival. The arbitrary nature of divine grace as understood in this way is offensive to the human soul and our commitment to justice. It is also inherently unreliable.

There always has been, and I suspect always will be, a tension, if not a contradiction, between the traditional Christian understanding of God and our common human experience. If you are paying attention at all you probably will already have fallen down on one side or the other. Many choose God, most commonly appealing to arguments about human free will (God can't, due to self-imposed restrictions, save the child because doing so would undermine human free will and thus the potential of and for the divine-human relationship) and arguments about God's mysterious ways (God won't save the child the reasons for which are never revealed and even if they were would be incomprehensible to human beings). There have been, no doubt, billions of words written and spoken articulating complex theological constructs explaining and justifying these two appeals. For others, however, the weight of nature's indifference, human brutality and injustice render any notion of God as illogical, irrational and offensive to human intelligence.

At this point some are accusing me of heresy and faithlessness and others of naiveté. I have no time for the judgment of the first group, but I do take the accusation of the second seriously. I believe the charge of naiveté is that I am being…What? I reject the words "childish" and "child-like" to describe my position because both imply that children lack intelligence and spiritual depth that they clearly possess. I also reject the word "primitive" because that implies that indigenous people were and are, well, childish or child-like (as rejected above) in their natural and spiritual interpretations of realty. This is clearly not the case. So, I will use the word "unsophisticated": I believe that the charge of naiveté accuses me of being unsophisticated in my understanding of and relationship with God and that my unsophistication assumes that the divine-human relationship is based on rewards and punishments.

In my defence: In order to make meaning in an indifferent universe, human beings impose on reality an ethical field that bestows moral meaning on all actions, and sometimes inactions, of sentient beings. If we assume that God is a sentient being and not just an unconscious Force, then it is not wrong to require God to embrace even a limited human understanding of ethics and morality (if God has a more sophisticated and just field of ethics, I'm all ears). To include God in a field of ethics is not to fall back on worshipping a God of rewards and punishments: I am moral because God will reward me and I am not immoral because God will punish me. We, and God, are not ethical because of what we can get and avoid. We are ethical because there is a *prima facie* value to the goodness of ethics. That is to say, moral behaviour is good in and of itself and needs no further justification (it goes without saying that to assert that ethics has *prima facie* value is not to say that the duties and virtues of ethics are self-evident). So, if I demand that God is ethical, I do so not because I anticipate receiving numerous goodies, but because being ethical is good. And what meaningful understanding of the Christian God would not include goodness. For Christians, God is good by definition, and while the notion of divine goodness may embrace more than ethics, it nonetheless must include ethics and morality.

Some might say that God is actually the ethical field of which I speak and that moral goodness is not superimposed on the universe but is the creative force that brought the universe into being, that reality is by its very nature literally good. Perhaps, but this does not make sense to me. It implies that a natural event like an earthquake or a disease like cancer have moral value. In what meaningful sense can you say that the death of a hundred thousand people due to an earthquake is good or evil in an ethical sense? In what sense is suffering with cancer good or evil?

Fundamentalists of all faith traditions claim that there is a causal link between natural disasters and disease and human behaviour, but that doesn't make it so. The natural universe is indifferent. It is not in and of itself ethical. Only sentience can be ethical. Nor does human moral behaviour determine what happens in nature.

I am aware that some people say that having cancer "is a gift," that is to say it is good. The best I can say is that it is possible that I might find meaning in the experience of having cancer that I would not have otherwise found without the cancer, but to say that cancer is good is non-sense in my understanding of reality.

There is a qualitative difference between the actions and character of sentient beings and the shifting of tectonic plates or the mutation of cells. There is a qualitatively moral difference between a god who causes suffering, for whatever reason, and a god who abhors suffering. I do not believe in a god who inflicts human beings with suffering to test their faith and/or grasp on reality. But if the god who abhors suffering is more reasonable and acceptable, then what do we do with the death of the child?

When it's all said and done, the sophisticated God is as powerless in the face of the natural universe as I am, and must be *truly* powerless. Faking powerlessness isn't good enough here. Otherwise, we are back to the unsophisticated God of reward and punishment and our rationalizations of free will and mysterious ways to justify the cruel death of innocence.

The best I can do with a powerless god is to at least give that god the chance that I give my wife, that is to be my friend and companion through my suffering and possible death. In other words, I can accept love. If I hesitate it is not because the ephemeral nature of God denotes weakness. Beauty is ephemeral and can still knock you over. But given that my wife is much more tangible (I can feel her holding me when I despair and hurt), the God-thing can be hard work - of course believers would call that hard work having faith. I must confess, however, that there is that unsophisticated voice within me that still asks if God, and it's *God* I'm talking about, is so powerless in the face of an indifferent universe, then what's the point? (Guilty as charged.)

As for me and the small child, if she dies of her cancer and I don't of mine, in this indifferent universe with a powerless God there is no reason for me to be offended or to feel guilty. I can mourn her death and celebrate my survival, but both are just the way it turned out to be. The universe is completely indifferent to my fate. It will not go out of its way to help me or to harm me. It will not notice my living or my dying. God, while perhaps wishing me no harm and being aware of my living or dying, is nonetheless powerless to change my fate. The indifferent universe and the powerless God cannot hold my hand when I'm in pain. They cannot wash the sheets and make the bed when I can't lift a feather. They cannot cook me a warm meal when I have no appetite. They cannot clean my body when I can't move and don't really care. They cannot whisper in my ear when I'm frightened. And they cannot say goodbye when it's time for my world to end. I surely must rely on those who love me, and perhaps even those who have, for whatever reason, a passing thought of my existence if only for a moment.

My George W. Bush Emotional Strategy for Coping with Dis-Ease

Cancer has no inherent value and I see no value in having cancer. If there are lessons to be learned, I would rather learn them in another way. If there is something to be gained, I would rather gain it through some other means. I, unlike cancer, do have value and live not to destroy but to create, though admittedly I do not always succeed in this fundamental ambition. The only good thing that can be said about cancer is that the killing of its host (that would be me) is a suicidal act. If I were to die of cancer, at least I would have the pleasure of knowing it would go with me to the grave. I am not glad I have cancer. It is neither a gift from God nor Fate nor The Force. It quite simply sucks.

I am not at war with my cancer. I am not a warrior by nature, though like everyone else in the world circumstances have from time to time necessitated that I fight. However, this doesn't seem like one of those times. Keeping positive, to me, is not a form of warfare. Nor is living healthily. Or drinking pomegranate juice and eating broccoli. I realise if I die of cancer, as opposed to taking my own life before it kills me, people will say things like "he fought until the end" and "he was such a fighter." But, honestly, I'm not sure that would be the case.

In truth, having cancer and seeking treatment is about handing your body, and perhaps your life, over to others, to experts with exotic knowledge and remarkable skills. It is handing yourself over to numerous powerful drugs and hard technologies made of steel and plastic. It is about making yourself radically vulnerable. These are the acts of a person hoping someone else will kill his or her enemy before it kills them. Yes, you can help, but the real theatre is the operating theatre or the radiotherapy theatre or the chemotherapy theatre. Our job is to lie down and either go to sleep or keep very still. Those are not the acts of a warrior.

Some days before my radical prostatectomy my wife asked me if I had cried yet. I said, no, I had a strategy. It was not an unfair question. I'm not embarrassed to say I am a fairly emotional person. I should have had a career on the stage because all too often I wring every amount of emotion out of a situation. However, in this case I felt I couldn't afford to let the emotions of fear have their way for even a moment, for to do so would render me unable to face what so many others have faced with dignity.

Fear of:

> Radical vulnerability (I say radical because how much more vulnerable can you get then letting one stranger place you in a deep sleep while another stranger cuts you open);
> Being cut open;
> The robot;
> The surgical team having a bad day;
> Dying;
> Waking up and making a fool of myself in some humiliating way;
> Pain;
> Being a bad patient when I know everyone else is a great patient.

To deal with these fears I had a strategy I called my George W. Bush Emotional Strategy for Coping with Dis-Ease. You can picture George W. in his flight jacket, which he never wore in war, telling the bad guys in Iraq to "bring it on!" Well, that was my strategy too, but my pumped-up machismo was not directed at bad guys or at my cancer. No, this macho outcry was directed at the technology and chemistry that was about to assault my body in order to save my life.

> Anaesthesia – Bring It On!
> Surgery – Bring It On!.
> Robot – Bring It On!
> Drugs – Bring It On!
> Pain – Bring It On!
> All you Impersonal Mechanical and Chemical Scary Beasts – Bring It On!
> Do Your Best!
> Is that All You've Got?!
> Ha! I Laugh in Your Face!!

Well, you get the idea. No vulnerability until the moment of complete vulnerability. Admittedly my strategy had its limits but it did get me to that small room lying on my back, with a tap in my wrist and sensors on my forehead, falling into a deep sleep without having to hide behind my metaphorical mother's metaphorical skirt.

It must be said, my wife was not completely convinced by my George W. Bush Emotional Strategy so instead gave me some new age crap about tears releasing toxins. I didn't buy it, but I did google tears and toxins when she wasn't looking. This is what I found: Emotional tears (as against tears caused, say, by hitting your thumb with a hammer) were found to contain approximately 24% more protein than reflex tears and had increased concentrations of prolactin, manganese, potassium and serotonin. Further, tears help you see better (not really important in my preparation for surgery), kill bacteria (could be useful), elevate mood (that would be good), lower stress (also good), release feelings (not good at all), and, yes, remove toxins (though some think the toxin thing is debatable). Having absorbed all this I went back to my wife and said something like this: I can't afford to cry before the surgery, but, and you can probably take this to the bank, sometime after the surgery, after I've returned home and the stress, pain and drugs kick in, I will no doubt release a seeming lifetime of toxins.

After two and a half days in the hospital I returned home on a Monday evening and went straight to bed. The dam burst the next morning. I hadn't taken a shower since Friday morning. We put a chair in the bathroom that I used to steady myself as I stepped into the tub. I couldn't touch my abdomen it was so sore, swollen and bruised. Even the water from the shower was unpleasant against my stomach. When I had finished washing I turned off the shower and stood while my wife handed me a towel. I could see my body in the mirror. I dried my upper body, stepped out of the tub leaning on the chair. My wife began to dry my legs and I began to cry quietly. I wasn't upset because I needed help drying my legs. I accepted that I needed help and would for the next week. It was the sight of my body in the mirror. It was ugly. The sight left me feeling extremely fragile. There were the wounds and the catheter in my penis attached to a wet leg bag. And I was in pain. I started to cry harder, shuffled to the bed and sat down. The crying became weeping and the weeping wailing. Just couldn't stop it. I cried like a baby.

To my wife, and to the entire universe if it cared to listen, I shouted, "I can't do this! I can't do this! I can't do this!" But while I was saying those words aloud, in my mind I was saying, "They cut me! They cut me! They cut me!"

And then I fell silent, the weeping became crying and the crying stopped as suddenly as it had begun.

The words are interesting. Even as I said "I can't do this" I knew very well I could, that indeed, I had no choice but to do it. I would live with the catheter, take pain medication and avoid touching my abdomen (and avoid mirrors). And yet I couldn't help saying it. Perhaps I was asking my wife for help, though I knew she had been nothing but helpful and would be until I was OK again. Or perhaps after the waiting, the surgery, the drugs, the horrible taxi ride home, the sleeplessness and the pain I was just soul weary and body exhausted and had to protest. As for the "They cut me!" Well, of course they cut me, I told them to cut me. I could have told them to radiate me, but I didn't. They did what I asked them to do, and apparently did it quite well. But still, to be cut, to look at your body and see seven sutured and bruised incisions was, at least for me, difficult.

But why the tears at that precise moment? I guess my George W. Bush Emotional Strategy had run its course on Tuesday morning as I stood dripping wet in front of a mirror. What I saw, dramatically speaking, was a wounded painful man who looked older than his years and utterly vulnerable to the pressures and knocks the universe would throw at him. A man too damn naked, and not a pretty sight I can tell you. He looked as if the slightest whisk of air, undetected by the most delicate of instruments, would knock him over. The stress, fear and drugs had had their way.

Perhaps it wasn't clever of me, the one who claims not to be a warrior, to choose a rich boy fraud of a warrior to be the inspiration of my emotional strategy. After I released all that protein, prolactin, manganese, potassium and serotonin, I can't say I felt less stressed and enjoyed elevated moods, though perhaps I did see better. But it seemed pretty clear that with all those toxins also went the last vestige of Bring It On macho posturing. My George W. Bush Emotional Strategy became bankrupt as the last tear dried. What followed were weeks of mood swings with the occasional "bad day." It wasn't the medication schedule or the pain that never quite disappeared. It wasn't the sleeplessness. It wasn't the dealing with the catheter, trying to avoid pulling or jerking the tube, the failure to do so being very unpleasant. It wasn't the emptying of the leg or night bag of urine or even the awkwardness of sitting on the toilet trying to defecate without pulling the catheter tube and stretching the opening of my offended penis. It was the having been run over by a train, the time needed to heal, the worry that something might yet go wrong that challenged my moods.

For those of you who might be facing what I have faced, I think the George W. Bush Emotional Strategy is not the best way forward. I have a dear friend living in New York City who thought he might instead have imagined a beautiful peaceful pastoral place where he could sit quietly and calm himself. This strategy might have more staying power, and given my experience of a rather limited strategy, I am now recommending the Beautiful Peaceful Pastoral Emotional Strategy for Coping with Dis-Ease. And to help that strategy along its way, a closing thought by Sharon Olds in her poem *Bruise Ghazal*:

Even as we speak, the work is being done, within. You were born to heal. [21]

The Things We Won't Talk About

David Foster Wallace argues in an essay that in sports there is a "kinetic beauty" which has universal appeal, that has nothing to do with cultural norms or sexual desires, but is apparently associated with "human beings' reconciliation with the fact of having a body."[22] Though Wallace's comments about beauty and sports are interesting, what intrigues me here is his comments about reconciliation. In a footnote he justifies his claim that we seek reconciliation with the fact of having bodies like this:

> There's a great deal that's bad about having a body. If this is not so obviously true that no one needs examples, we can just quickly mention pain, sores, odors, nausea, aging, gravity, sepsis, clumsiness, illness, limits – every last schism between our physical wills and our actual capacities. Can anyone doubt we need help being reconciled? [23]

Well, when you put it that way, he's right, even though it does remind us of the unhelpful Descartian dualism between mind (spirit/soul if you prefer) and body, the very dualism that postmodernism tried to argue into nonexistence. [24] Unfortunately, when our bodies let us down, it's hard not to see ourselves as two entities needing reconciliation. It is possible that in the case of prostate cancer and treatment it's the very failure to reconcile ourselves with our bodies' burdens that makes it difficult for us to talk about what is going on. Not only have our bodies become unpleasant and perhaps painful, they have also become damn bothersome and embarrassing.

Both my grandfather and father had prostate cancer so the possibility of my contracting the disease had been on my radar for quite some time. Needless to say, I didn't beat the odds. At around forty years old I started asking men who had had treatment for prostate cancer what the deal was. No one would answer my questions, either evading or simply refusing to talk about what was happening to them. Reading about prostate problems and the consequences of treatments is vitally important, but hearing first hand from someone experiencing those consequences is something else entirely.

As I approached my radical prostatectomy, and having read about the likely consequences, I found that both anticipated embarrassment and the unarticulated fear of being estranged from my body occupied my mind (again, and for the last time, soul or spirit if you prefer). I was embarrassed to walk into a chemist and buy adult diapers and pads, and was relieved to see self-checkout kiosks. (As it turned out, I didn't buy my diapers and pads because I wasn't sure what I would need, which was a good move. The NHS gave me a large supply of diapers and pads the day I had my catheter removed). But more important than my embarrassment was the concern, on some days fear, that I would have to learn how to live with a new unpleasant and dysfunctional body. In Wallace's words, I feared I would have difficulty reconciling myself to the fact that I had a troublesome body.

So, the things we won't talk about. Here's the low down as I see it.

With most treatments for prostate cancer men will experience incontinence. As I used to say to my wife before I researched the issue, I feared I would spend the rest of my life pissing in my pants. There was something profoundly embarrassing about the idea of "being reduced" to needing diapers because I wouldn't be able to "control myself." And there was also something profoundly disturbing about having a body that I might not be able to control on such a basic and sensitive level. As it turned out, my fears were misplaced.

Men will more than likely experience both *urge incontinence* and *stress incontinence*. The first is the feeling of suddenly having to urinate followed by a bladder contraction and involuntary loss of urine. The second is leakage of urine when you stand or sit, cough, lift something, etc.[25] Loss of control through urine flow and leakage is unpleasant, but the statistics are encouraging. Depending on who you read and/or talk to, only 3% to 5% of men will experience severe incontinence after six months, and most men regain control of their bladders within three months.[26] To ensure you are among the 95% to 97% of men who do regain control, you must do your pelvic floor exercises, also called Kegel exercises. A quote from Johns Hopkins might encourage you:

> In one study, 68% of men who did Kegel exercises after radical prostatectomy regained urinary continence within 3 months, compared with 37% of men who did not do these exercises.[27]

Your oncology nurse or doctor will tell you about how to do the exercises but there are numerous websites on the Internet that you can explore. The technique is the same no matter where you look, but the frequency of doing the exercises will vary. I was told by one source to do them once an hour, by another five times a day and by yet another three times a day. I do them four times a day.

When I had my catheter removed my oncology nurse told me the first few days would be the worst and I would need to wear diapers after which I could move to using pads in my underwear. Actually, I moved to pads on the second day. Interestingly, once the catheter was removed and I stood in front of the nurse pulling on my man-diaper, I wasn't embarrassed at all (and a lot of the credit goes to my nurse who handled the situation well). It was not my fault I got cancer. Incontinence is a result of treatment not a failure of character. I had to use diapers and pads, so get over it. I would do my exercises. None of this had anything to do with my integrity or dignity. It was just bloody life. I didn't, in the end, feel like I had been reduced to an infant or had advanced in time to a smelly decrepit old man.

I must confess, however, that reconciling myself to this new, and I was hoping temporary, body was at times difficult. At first I was hesitant to go to dinner with my wife on our regular Friday night outing to the local Italian restaurant (hesitant, that was, until she rather firmly reminded me that she had spent years of her life using pads for menstrual bleeding and still went out to dinner with me!). When I felt down, I did an extra round of pelvic floor exercises. And as my wife told me, I had already once in my life learned to control my bladder and I could do it again (it took me a minute to understand). Still, my emotions were all over the place and in the first five weeks after having the catheter removed I experienced some depressing days. My point being, don't get depressed about having depressing days.

There is a good chance that during the first month or so after your catheter is removed you will pass with your urine what my oncology nurse called "debris," which for me was varying sizes of black flakes. Most were tiny, but some I could feel passing through my urethra. I was not told about this by anyone, and while not shocking, it was worrying simply because I didn't know what it was. As it turns out, it is fairly common. My passing of debris lasted for about four weeks. I was told not to worry but to drink plenty of liquids to make sure the urethra did not "clog up."

There is one more issue around urination, however, and that is *bladder retention*. We spend all our time worrying about pissing in our pants, but also must be concerned about being able to piss at all. During surgery the urethra is cut and then sutured back to the base of the bladder. It is possible that scar tissue will form in the urethra and eventually restrict the flow of urine. Unfortunately, scar tissue develops slowly and can take from one to two years before impacting urinary flow. In my case, my flow has been erratic, some days worrying and other days fairly normal (it always seemed to me it should be one way or the other!). The medical world treats this kind of bladder retention rather lightly, meaning it is usually a “minor procedure” to make things right. But for me, and I suspect for most men, I’m hoping I can avoid having a camera jammed into my penis, scar tissue scraped away, stents inserted, and whatever else the medical experts do. If you do need to have your urethra cleared of scar tissue, you may then also need to pull your diapers and pads out of the closet. The procedure can lead to loss of bladder control. One man I spoke to suffered incontinence so badly after the procedure he finally had to have an artificial urethral sphincter implanted to control his flow. Happily it worked. Bottom line, however, if you develop bladder retention you will know it and you will have to seek medical help.

As we know, a man’s penis has two functions and both are affected by prostate cancer treatment. You can be assured you will experience *erectile dysfunction.* Radical prostatectomy, external beam radiotherapy, brachytherapy, high intensity focused ultrasound (HIFU) and cryotherapy can all damage the nerves and blood vessels that are necessary for an erection.

I can’t remember how many times I have been asked about my “erectile history” in the past six months. When I tell them I had never experienced erectile dysfunction they have always said that was good because it increased my chances of having erections in the future. However, in my pre-op interview with the surgeon he also said I would probably never have the same quality of erections after the surgery (I found the pre-op interview positive, helpful and sensitive, but very much more realistic than other conversations up to that point).

Since puberty I have been having an average of four spontaneous erections each night (or so I assume because I was to told that is the average for the average male). From my teens on sexual intercourse has been a source of pleasure and an important means of communicating intimacy and love. As I anticipated my surgery, I found that I could not quite grasp who I would be without the ability to get an erection. I realise I'm on thin ice here, the thinnest of the ice depending upon how well I can articulate what I felt, thought and experienced. Some very dear feminist friends might already be thinking about men being led by their penises or thinking with their dicks. But the truth is, I am a male, I have a penis and get, well got, erections every day of my life. Who the hell would I be without erections? Without making love? Without masturbation? Without those sometimes annoying and sometime opportune morning spontaneous erections? What and who is a man with long term erectile dysfunction? What does he do with his libido, because treatment does not affect that (nor does it affect your ability to have orgasms, though with an important difference – more about that later)? So, you can still get turned on, but you can't get it up. What the hell is that about?! You have to laugh.[28]

Here's how it works:

> The penis is made up of nerves, smooth muscle, and blood vessels. Within the penis are two cylindrical chambers – called the corpora cavernosa, or corporal bodies – that extend from the base to the tip. When a man has an erection, smooth muscle tissue within the penis relaxes, causing these spongy chambers to dilate and fill with blood. The swollen corporal bodies press against and close the veins that normally allow blood to flow away from the penis; as a result, the penis remains engorged with blood. After orgasm, the smooth muscle tissue contracts, and blood once again exits the penis.
>
> This process is initiated by signals passing through nerve bundles that run along both sides of the prostate toward the penis. Radical prostatectomy can lead to erectile dysfunction if one or both of these nerve bundles is damaged during surgery. Nerve damage does not affect sensation in the penis, but it does impair a man's ability to achieve a normal erection. Radiation treatment also can result in erectile dysfunction by damaging these nerve bundles or the arteries

that carry blood to the penis.[29]

Even if your surgeon practices nerve-sparing surgery, but that does not mean you will not have problems. (If you're having a prostatectomy you should ask your surgeon if he or she practices nerve-sparing surgery.) My oncology nurse put me on erectile medications soon after my catheter was removed, but warned me that there would be little or no effect for some time. My GP, always honest with me, said: "This can take forever." The statistics here are less encouraging than those for incontinence. Again, do your own research and talk to your doctor and nurse, but what I've read and been told is that 40% to 50% of men will regain erectile function within the first year and 30% to 60% within the first two years (looking at the other side of those coins is a bit depressing). I've also been told regaining erectile function may take up to five years.

In the past the medical profession has been accused of not taking the issue of erectile dysfunction seriously (interesting since I assume in the past most of the surgeons were men). Now the experts are as positive as they can be and even refuse to use the word impotence. It is now a matter of dysfunction and function. If you experience long term dysfunction, or if you are just impatient (for which I can't blame you) there are numerous possibilities. Here is a list I have taken from Prostate Cancer UK:

Life Style - diet and exercise;

Tablets - most common are Viagra® (sildenafil), Cialis® (tadalafil), Levitra® (fardenafil);

Injections - injecting alprostadi into the base of the penis;

Pellets - alprostadi in pellet form is inserted into the penis with an applicator (a plunger), the penis is then massaged to melt the pellet;

Vacuum Pump and a Rubber Ring (Cock Ring) – kind of obvious, but put your penis in a cylinder, pump and draw blood into the penis and put the cock ring around the base of your penis to block the blood from retreating;

Surgical Implants – There are two basic types of implants: a semi-

> rigid rod that keeps your penis relatively hard all the time but is bendable when you are not having sex; and an inflatable implant with a pump in the scrotum, squeeze the pump and the inflatable implant is filled with a saline fluid. [30]

All these treatments have varying degrees of success, and to be honest a few of them would take some getting used to.

As I said above, treatment for prostate cancer does not affect your libido or your ability to have an orgasm. However, if you have radiotherapy or brachytherapy you may produce less semen and thus your ejaculation will be diminished. But, if you have radical prostatectomy you will never ejaculate again (and it goes without saying you will be infertile). Here's why:

> Sperm is produced in the testicles and transported through tubes to the prostate gland. Semen, the solution that carries sperm, is produced by both the prostate gland and the seminal vesicles, glands attached to the prostate. Prior to ejaculation, tubes from the testicles carry sperm to the prostate, where sperm mixes with semen. This fluid is then ejaculated during orgasm by a connection to the urethra called the ejaculatory ducts.
>
> After ejaculation, the nerves stop sending messages, the smooth muscle contracts, blood flow to the penis is reduced, the veins loosen their hold so blood can leave the penis and the erection fades away. [31]

During surgery the seminal vesicles and the ejaculatory ducts are removed with the prostate gland. No vesicles and ducts, no ejaculations. For some men this is no big deal and for others it's a deal breaker as far as surgery is concerned. For me, the two obvious treatments given my medical history were surgery and radiotherapy and I wanted the cancer out of my body. In other words, I was willing to deal with the need to be reconciled to the fact that I had a body that no longer ejaculated during orgasm. I should confess that anticipating a new me is not the same thing as living with a new me, and now that the deed has been done I'm finding the adjustment slightly more difficult than I anticipated. However, I'll live.

That's the down and dirty from a guy who is going through it. But again I must repeat, I have had no medical training, so do your own reading and talk to the medical experts.

My dad, bless his heart, could never talk to me about what he was going through post surgery. His embarrassment of and alienation from his body simply shut him down. That's OK, though it would have been nice to have talked about it. As for me, for whatever reason, I have no difficulty talking about the consequences of prostate cancer treatment. It's no fun, it can be difficult, but in that mind/body split, none of this says anything about my integrity of being. It does say a lot about my willingness and ability to be reconciled to the fact that I am inexorably a physical being.

Lights and Tunnels

I may be fortunate. It may be that the light at the end of my personal tunnel is sunshine and not an oncoming train. My final pathology report was excellent. My first post-op PSA reading was excellent. I'm recovering well from surgery. My incontinence is already an unpleasant dream. My body is forgetting the brutal invasion of technology and chemistry. The seven scars are beginning to fade. The pain is gone, and because my body cannot remember its intensity, the pain has moved from experience to idea. My mind is forgetting how vulnerable radical vulnerability is, and here too the experiential becomes the conceptual. I worried, I feared, I wept, but there is no angst now. As it should be. (Admittedly when it comes to erections my penis is still on strike, but negotiations continue, and not without hope. And it may be another year or two before I know if I will experience bladder retention due to the build up of scar tissue in my urethra and thus need further unpleasant treatment.)

Again I quote my favourite poet Sharon Olds: "You were born to heal."[32]

Still, I say I may be fortunate because I guess you really never know about cancer, the bastard. Why else would the medical folk be checking my PSA for the rest of my life? There is a chance, slim though it may be, that no matter how excellent things appear to be, cancer is nonetheless lingering somewhere unnoticed, waiting and wanting to commit suicide and take me with it. And yet if I am honest with myself, it is more than likely sunshine rather than disaster I see ahead. So, when it's all said and done, I am a happy boy, with only a slight shadowy qualification. The trick now is to stop worrying and simply live (which is different from living simply).

Unfortunately, at least for me, *simply* living can be complicated. Simply living implies that I should live with the minimum of existential angst, that I should take it easy, perhaps even chill! That I should simply appreciate and value life. But hey...

Simple:

Clear;
Pure;
Unambiguous;

Easy.

Easy:

Simple;
Effortless;
Painless;
Light.

Ease:

The condition of being comfortable or relieved;
Freedom from pain, worry, or agitation;
Freedom from constraint or embarrassment;
Naturalness;
Freedom from difficulty, hardship, or effort.

How often have we heard people who have faced death or are facing death say that they have a heightened awareness of and value for life? Surely that is, at least in part, living simply and easily. Unfortunately for some of us, there is another side to that particular coin, which is not to say that it is the dark side or the negation of the other. It is rather to say that we can possess both easy unambiguous appreciation and complicated heavy anxiety at the same time. We human beings are gifted with and sometimes burdened by consciousness, which often leads to both ethical and metaphysical pondering. Any major disease can certainly disturb both the physical and mental *ease* with which we hope to live. I can at the same time appreciate in new ways my living *and* wonder what the hell my life now means. I can both celebrate *and* deliberate (or even de-liberate[33]).

So, given all that, and now that the light is getting brighter as I near the end of my tunnel, what's on my mind?

While for me the colours may not be more colourful and the music more musical, I'm damned thrilled that this particular cancer didn't get me.

If you are about to go through or are actually going through what I went through, I hope you have a spouse, partner, family member, or friend to go through it with you. I had my wife, and while we experienced things differently, it must be said that her living was also without ease for a long time. Still, she was there for the worry, hope, boredom, anxiety, pain, embarrassment, agitation, trauma, healing and relief. It had been a long time since we were so focused on each other, particularly during that first week at home after surgery. But be warned. Life must return to normal. When this focus in the moment of crisis ends, you will know it. When my wife returned to work at the beginning of the second week at home, I not only missed the attention she gave me, and it would be disingenuous not to admit that, I also missed the intensity of being us. The with-you-no-matter-what. The with-you-all-the-way-to-the-end-whether-that-is-healing-or-dying. When that kind of being with you ends, you may feel abandoned for a few days. It will pass.

I owe a lot, perhaps my life, to my GP, ward nurses, speciality nurses, anaesthetist, urologist, oncology nurse, oncologist and surgeons.[34] It's hard to imagine they could have been much better. And though the current coalition government in the UK would have us believe the NHS is in crisis in order to justify their major top-down "reforms," which in reality are the fulfilment of the Tory dream of privatising the service (aided by the Liberal Democrat Party), healthcare in crisis was not what I experienced. And in addition to the NHS was, and still is, Prostate Cancer UK, good people doing good work.

I underestimated the emotional impact of the whole experience, from diagnosis through recovering at home to discovering the new normal of my life. On the day I received my final pathology I was thrilled with the good news. But three days later I became depressed and it lasted for a couple of weeks. I have no idea where it came from and found it hard to talk about. I could talk about incisions, diapers, catheters, erections and pissing in my pants, but I could not talk about this unpleasant energy sapping mystery. A good friend sent me an email saying it was not uncommon for people to become depressed after major surgery, and while the information did not flick the appropriate switch, it did help. Most importantly, eventually, the depression passed. However, if you experience the same, talk to someone.

I'm not to blame. Prostate cancer is a disease that at best disrupts and at worse kills. It was not my fault, and it is not yours. It just is. So, you can imagine I was thrilled to read in the paper the other day that studies show cancer, including prostate cancer, is not caused by stress at work, for example.[35] That means, while you shouldn't blame yourself, you cannot blame your boss.

A few days before my radical prostatectomy I read *Mortality* by Christopher Hitchens.[36] Perhaps it was not the most clever thing I've ever done. The book is Hitchens' account of dying of cancer. But I wanted to be reminded of the severity of what I faced – Cancer! And I wanted to hear how someone with intelligence, humour and dignity faced his dis-ease. I would like to say I laughed in the face of Death. However, in all honesty when I contemplated the darker of the possibilities that lay before me, I was scared shitless. Believe it or not, *Mortality* helped me.

Finally, I'm changed. I don't yet know how much or in what ways. I feel the figuring it out coming on and there's no sense in standing in its way. And I guess the figuring will be done in the light.

---

[1] See: http://oxforddictionaries.com/definition/english/disease.

[2] See: http://healing.about.com/od/energyhealing/g/dis-ease.htm.

[3] See: http://dictionary.reference.com/browse/dis-.

[4] I've read that to date approximately 27 molecular varieties of prostate cancer have been found. However, Dr. Kate Holmes of Prostate Cancer UK says that scientists believe 27 molecular varieties is probably "the tip of the iceberg."

[5] Hitchens, Christopher. *Mortality*. London: Atlantic Books, 2012, p. 90.

[6] By "meditations" I am not implying what I wrote is concerned with transcendental meditation or even religious deliberation. I am more interested in the word's meaning as a written or spoken discourse expressing well thought-out opinions on a subject; or thinking deeply about an area of concern. And I confess, I am simply weary of the word "reflections."

[7] My main sources are: Carter, H. Ballentine, *The Johns Hopkins White Papers: Prostate Disorders*, 2006; Marks, Sheldon, *Prostate & Cancer: A Family Guide to Diagnosis, Treatment, and Survival*, Cambridge MA: Da Capo Press, 2009; the Prostate Cancer Charity UK *Tool Kit* and website, 2013; lectures at the Royal Free London NHS Foundation Trust, 2012 and 2013 (organised by the oncology department); and discussions with my GP Dr. Barbara Frosh and with doctors and nurses at the Royal Free London NHS Foundation Trust and the University College London Hospitals NHS Foundation Trust.

[8] Allen, Woody. *Love and Death*. United Artist, 1975.

[9] Bright, William. *A Coyote Reader*. Berkeley: University of California Press, 1993, p. 31.

[10] Ibid., pp. 87-88.

[11] Prostate Cancer UK: http://prostatecanceruk.org/.

[12] I have spoken to men who found the procedure very painful.

[13] See: Carter, H. Ballentine, *The Johns Hopkins White Papers: Prostate Disorders*, 2006.

[14] To my claim that men don't like things being jammed down their penises, a friend in New York City emailed: "I will say, though, that as for men putting things in their penises, there is a practice among gay men (I don't know about heteropractices) of putting rods down their shaft. It's called "sounding," and it is sometimes done with electrical stimulation to the metal rod. I hear it's quite stimulating. I'll believe the reports, not about to try it out on myself. Sales are great, if you go online to Mr. S. Leathers and hunt around in the sex toys for sounding equipment. And there you'll see it, maybe even with a picture. If you can't find a photo, just to see that not all men wince at the idea of something shoved into their penis, I'll find one for you."
If gay men are "sounding," I suspect straight men are too.

[15] Gutierrez, Gustavo. *On Job: God-Talk and the Suffering of the Innocent*. New York: Orbis Books, 1989.

[16] Ibid., p. 1.

[17] See: Dictionary.com: http://dictionary.reference.com/browse/Disinterested.

[18] In a robotic assisted radical prostatectomy, your body is placed with your head lower than your feet. After four or five hours in this position your eyes, face and brain can become swollen. The swelling of the brain can cause confusion.

[19] If you are unfamiliar with the Star Trek universe and the evil Borg go to:
http://www.startrek.com/database_article/borg.

[20] Normally I would have seen both the day after surgery. However, my surgery was on a Friday afternoon and so I was attended to by the staff on duty for that particular weekend.

[21] Olds, Sharon. *Stag's Leap*. New York: Alfred A. Knopf, 2012, p.67.

[22] Wallace, David Foster. *Both Flesh and Not*. London: Hamish Hamilton, 2012.

[23] Ibid., p. 8.

[24] The problem of mind and matter, or consciousness and the brain, was addressed by René Descartes in the 17th Century, resulting in Cartesian dualism. Descartes identified the mind with consciousness and "distinguished this from the brain as the seat of intelligence. Hence, he was the first to formulate the mind-body problem in the form in which it exists today." For a brief overview see:

http://en.wikipedia.org/wiki/Dualism_%28philosophy_of_mind%29.

[25] Carter, H. Ballentine. *The Johns Hopkins White Papers: Prostate Disorders*, 2006, pp 63-64.

[26] Do check these stats out for yourself. My main sources are: Carter, H. Ballentine, *The Johns Hopkins White Papers: Prostate Disorders*, 2006; Marks, Sheldon, *Prostate & Cancer: A Family Guide to Diagnosis, Treatment, and Survival*, Cambridge MA: Da Capo Press, 2009; the Prostate Cancer Charity UK *Tool Kit* and website, 2013; lectures at the Royal Free London NHS Foundation Trust, 2012 (organised by the oncology department).

[27] Carter, H. Ballentine. op. cit., pp 64.

[28] I realise all these questions are not the end of the world and are answerable, but to dismiss them as just male penis concerns is not realistic. To most men, our penises, erections, orgasms and our ability to have intercourse are very important.

[29] Carter, H. Ballentine. op. cit., pp 67-68.

[30] Prostate Cancer UK: http://prostatecanceruk.org/.

[31] UPMC Cancer Center: http://www.upmccancercenter.com/cancer/prostate/erectiledysfunction.html.

[32] Olds, Sharon. loc.cit.

[33] The prefix “de” means to do or make the opposite of; reverse. See: http://www.thefreedictionary.com/de-.

[34] My excellent GP is Dr. Barbara Frosh. My local hospital where most of my care was done is Royal Free London NHS Trust. The hospital where my radical prostatectomy and immediate care was done is University College London Hospitals NHS Trust. Prostate Cancer UK, provided me with both written material in the form of the *Tool Kit* (all the information you want to know about prostate cancer and treatments) and personal advice from the specialist nurses on the telephone. The link to PCUK is http://prostatecanceruk.org/.

[35] Boseley, Sarah. Health Editor *The Guardian*, “Stress at work unlikely to trigger common cancer, say researchers,” 7 February 2013. See: http://www.guardian.co.uk/society/2013/feb/07/stress-work-not-trigger-cancer. The Guardian article is based on a report by the British Medical Journal, “Work stress and risk of cancer; meta-analysis of 5700 incident cancer events in 116000 European men and women,” BMJ 2012; 346 doi: http://dx.doi.org/10.1136/bmj.f165, Published 7 February 2013.

[36] Hitchens, Christopher. *Mortality*. London: Atlantic Books. 2012.

www.ingramcontent.com/pod-product-compliance
Lightning Source LLC
LaVergne TN
LVHW041252150826
845673LV00008B/2558

* 9 7 9 8 5 0 7 0 7 1 9 5 1 *